Zen

and the

Art of Nursing

Susan L. Schoenbeck, MSN, RN

Book production and editing by
Springwaterpress.com, Oregon City, Oregon

Website by ecentech.com

As I sat down to review Zen and the Art of Nursing, I was unsure what I would find. While I know nursing well through my 46 years as a nurse, I know only a little about Zen. But the title intrigued me - and I was curious.

What I found was a fascinating book but not just for reading - it provoked slowing down, reflecting, recalling old experiences and examining new patterns. Through the well-crafted, simple statements, I found myself learning about Zen and gaining an even deeper appreciation for nursing. I read certain passages and then stopped and appreciated the similarities. I read other passages and gained insights into my own behavior. The readings reminded me of the extraordinarily special relationships we nurses can have with our patients and their families, and the differences that we can make. But the readings also reminded me that we have to come fully open and prepared as we engage in these relationships. The investment is so worthwhile to our patients, their families and ourselves.

–Joanne Disch, PhD, RN, FAAN
Professor ad Honorem, University of Minnesota School of Nursing

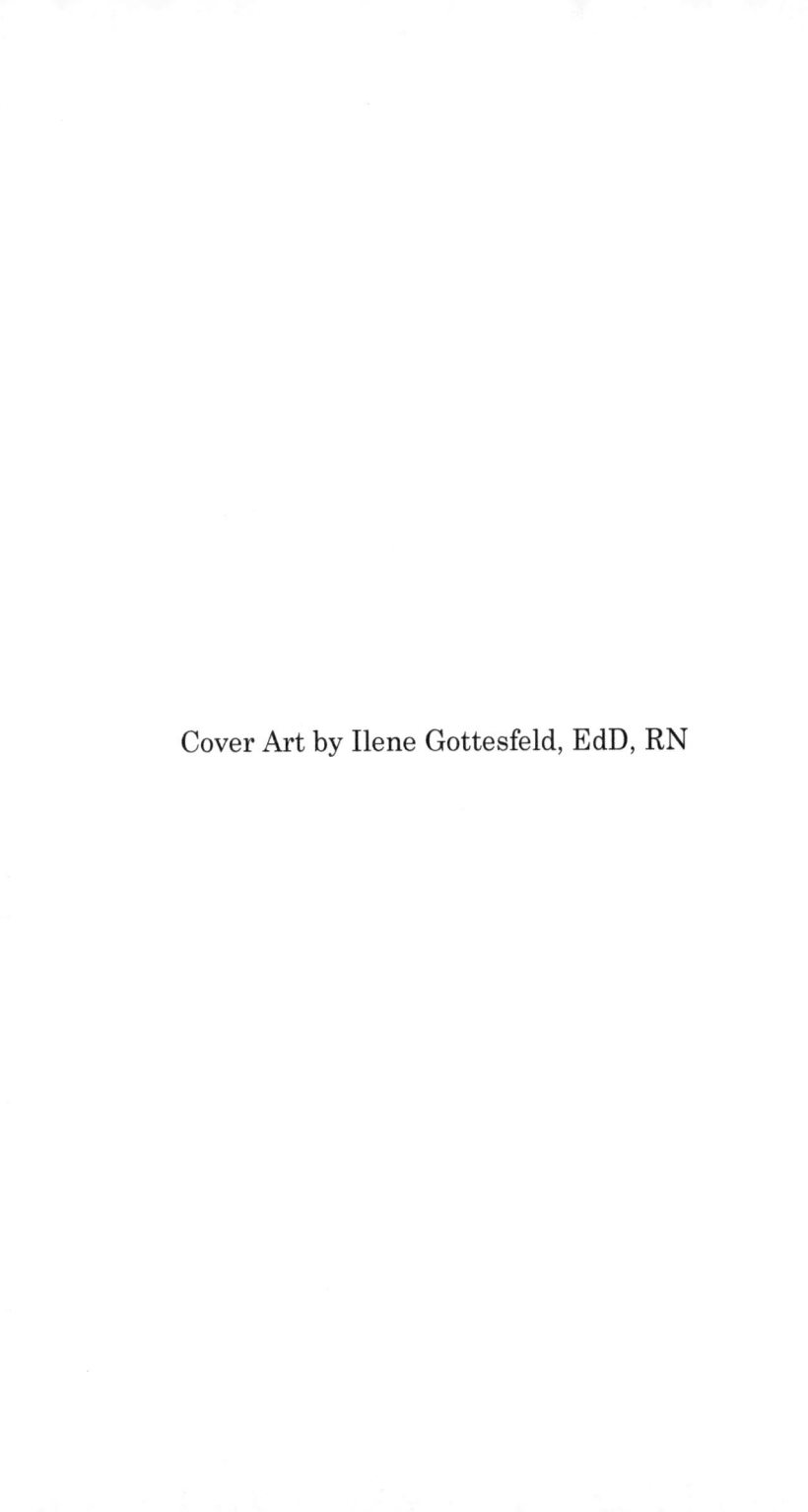

Cover Art by Ilene Gottesfeld, EdD, RN

Zen and the Art of Nursing

This book describes basic Zen. It provides readers with meditations that link Zen philosophy to nursing practices.

We Western-trained nurses often have trouble putting into words what it is we do for our clients besides the obvious carrying out of medical practitioner orders. In simplest terms, nurses may follow pathways not often walked before, weaving their healing presence into the lives of others. In other words, we Zen it!

There are many similarities between our best nursing practices and Zen, which began in China during the 6th century as a way of looking at the world with a centered and calm mind. Although associated with Buddhism, Zen is not a religion, but a meditative state linked to the search for truth and self-improvement. The meditations that follow will unlock new doors of perception and cultivate your Zen nature.

❖ Zen asks that we be quiet and contemplative at times, allowing surrounding energy forces to enter us.

- ❖ Zen tells us to be open to serendipity, releasing ourselves to the ebb and flow of daily life.

- ❖ Zen asks that we pay attention to the everyday moments of life.

- ❖ Zen encourages us to fully experience and appreciate each moment... one at a time.

- ❖ Zen underscores our true nature as one of compassion and wisdom.

- ❖ Zen instructs us that recognizing our own weaknesses and strengths helps us better understand the trials and tribulations of others.

- ❖ Zen teaches us that reflection on our own lives helps us realize not only how we can be better human beings, but also how we can help others to become kinder and gentler.

- ❖ Zen beholds the holy faces of the weak, the sick and the poor as representations of divine opportunity to serve in a secular world.

❖ Zen provides an even keel, rocking us gently, in life and death situations.

Many times nurses are listeners whose ears are fine-tuned to pick up on patients' innermost thoughts. A nurse's quiet presence creates a shared, safe space where humans can utter their most terrifying thoughts and most shamed actions without worry of being judged. From nurses, clients gain an acceptance that brings peacefulness that often cannot be explained with words, but is realized by the nurse and patient.

Countless times healing takes place in ways unknown to us when we operate from Zen-like state of being. That we cannot always grasp how this healing occurs makes such healing events no less significant.

The following meditations celebrate the interaction of nurses with their patients. These experiences often fall into the category of events that are beyond words, and remind us that each movement we make is full of potential and can be rich in rewards.

The Artists of Being Alive

The most visible creators I

know are those artists

whose medium is life itself.

The ones who express the inexpressible

without brush, hammer, clay or guitar.

They neither paint nor sculpt.

Their medium is being.

Whatever their presence touches

has increased life.

They see and do not have to draw.

They are the artists of being alive.

J. Stone

Looking Beyond Masks

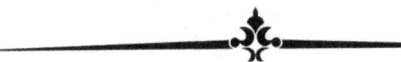

Zen is a way of looking at and through events. Patients are just like other people. They send out messages about who they say they are, who others think they are, and who they really are. Nurses look beyond the masks people wear and come to know who the patient is and what he or she needs most.

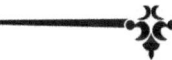

Asking

Zen has no map or destination. Zen encourages people to forge their own pathway of learning to better understand themselves and others. Nurses often do not know where their questions may lead. Despite not knowing, a nurse is comfortable searching for deeper meanings, thereby bringing better patient outcomes.

Being

In the mind of a nurse, a patient can be neither good nor bad. Such a distinction is artificial. People just "are." Nurses demonstrate that they can transcend circumstances, and work beside patients no matter what situations have brought them together.

Here and Now

Nurses meet patients whether they are:

- ✧ angry
- ✧ confused
- ✧ scared
- ✧ tired
- ✧ unsure
- ✧ recovering
- ✧ hopeful or hopeless

A patient's state of mind is never unexpected. The nurse explores, not ignores, the here-and-now feelings of a patient.

Teaching

Zen says teachers will appear
according to the learner's needs.
Nurses meet patients lost in a
labyrinth of unfamiliar places and
technologies. Nurses perform nursing
cares until such a time the patient or
other caregiver can take over the tasks.
Nurses are some of the best teachers.

Enlightenment

A nurse is enlightened through experiences with patients. Each patient causes the nurse to ask, "What is the reason I am here today?" The nurse finds wisdom from reflection on experiences with ordinary people who face extraordinary times.

Knowledge as a Key

Nurses understand that new knowledge comes their way daily. Each patient and each situation bring different lessons. To meet individual patient needs, nurses cobble together what they know from books and what they know from clinical experience into a practice that is both art and science. A nurse's expertise grows through practice.

Always Asking

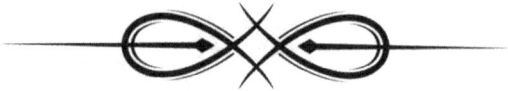

Zen does not hold all the answers. Zen urges us to continually question. Nurses are always asking patients questions. Nurses compare what the patient says with how the patient looks. They look for objective clues about how patients are really doing, not just how they say they are doing. Asking, looking and seeking answers always bring better results for patients.

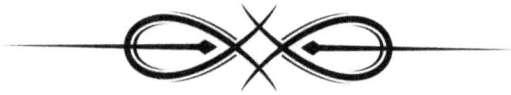

Digging for Meaning

Nurses understand that sometimes patients will say "yes" when they mean "no," just to be nice. Nurses have the good sense not to believe everything they hear, but to dig deeper than asking a "yes or no" question. Nurses ask patients to tell their stories to find out what really is on their minds. Digging for meaning, rather than settling for pleasantries, uncovers truth. "Tell me" are powerful words in a nurse's vocabulary.

The Many Paths to Truth

Zen teaches us our ways of living are not the only ones that may lead to truth and beauty. Nurses meet people from all walks of life, and from varied cultures, religions and social statuses. Because nurses understand all ways of knowing are important, they do not show bias for one way of life over another. Nurses understand patients who take other paths, and respect their journeys.

Zen Is About Real Life

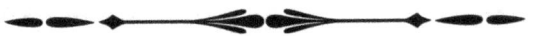

Nurses live ordinary lives extraordinarily well. To comfort, to bathe, to soothe, to listen...these are daily acts of nurses. Nurses are extraordinary at doing ordinary acts of kindness.

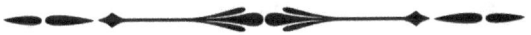

Faith to Follow

Zen makes no promise of Heaven.
Likewise, nurses are assured of no
great reward for their services. But like
the followers of Zen, nurses understand
that what they do is of importance not
only to the people they serve but to
their own journey of self-improvement
and self-discovery.

Getting Started Each Day

Zen does not tell us how long our journey will be. But Zen urges us to get started. Nurses begin each new shift not knowing what will transpire. Nursing is not a job for those who are passive. Nurses don't mind facing the unknown. They understand each day is part of a greater journey.

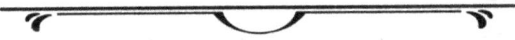

The Simple Life

Zen tells us we find what is important
in the simple life. Nurses wade through
a lot of paperwork and bureaucracy to
get to the really important task of
interacting with patients in miraculous
ways. Nurses seek the simple life,
where clear communication with
patients is priority.

Peacefulness

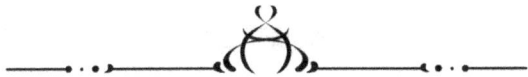

Zen teaches us inner peace makes you peaceful on the outside. Many times nurses have to take deep breaths and pull energy and strength from within to carry out complex procedures that are uncomfortable for patients, in order to advance wellness.

Dialogue

Zen leads us on the path toward dialogue. Ethical behavior occurs when people on both sides of an issue come to an agreement on what action is best. Nurses help patients and their family members dialogue on important issues.

Dignity

Dignity matters. Nurses protect the
privacy of patients. The art of nursing
is based on a framework of caring and
a respect for human dignity.

Comfort

Zen knows there are no points given in
the next world for suffering. Nurses work
hard to understand what time of the day
and night pain comes to a patient. Nurses
determine where the pain is, what
activity precedes it, what aggravates the
pain, and what relieves the pain.
Comforting is a nursing art and practice.

Recognition

Zen sees no red or black skin, yellow or
white skin, or any in-between skin. Zen
recognizes the human spirit. Nurses
see beyond the earthly garments
people wear. Nurses recognize true
beings in need of care.

Waiting

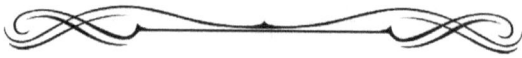

Zen teaches us that life will not wait
for us. We must travel the road now.
Nurses have many demands placed on
them each minute of their workday.
Nurses learn to sort through and act on
what is most important to those
waiting for nursing care.

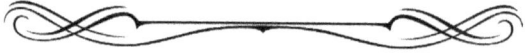

The Moment

Zen teaches us to live in the moment.
Nurses identify critical moments in
patients' lives. The actions nurses take
in those moments make differences in
patients' well-being.

Pride

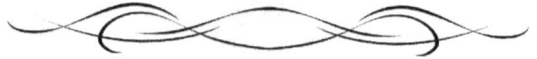

Zen reminds us we are all brothers and sisters. Nurses do not let pride stop them from working side-by-side with team members that have opinions different from their own. Nurses work hand-in-hand to create the greatest good for patients.

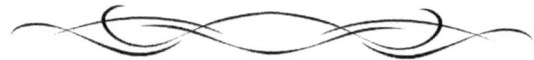

Reverence

Zen followers revere the universe.
Nurses understand that patients are
the center of their work universe.
Nurses respectfully show attention to
patients' concerns.

One Thing at a Time

Zen asks us to focus on one thing at a
time. In this hectic world, nurses
consciously put aside thoughts of all
that must be done to dwell quietly with
a patient for one moment in time.

Receptive

Followers of Zen know that it is often
important to separate from what is
going on in the world to concentrate on
what is happening to the patient.
Nurses learn how to shut out the rest
of the world to be receptive to only one
person...the patient.

Mind Talk

Zen teaches us how to touch each other
with our minds. Sometimes the nurse
sits quietly beside a patient. When
close together in silence, the patient
understands the nurse cares deeply.

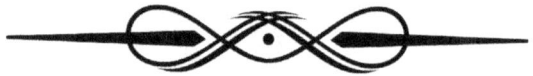

Finding the Way

To find your way, you must sometimes close your eyes, relying on your mind to guide you. When patients are unable to tell nurses what their problems are, nurses often must rely on their intuition to determine what best to do.

Silence

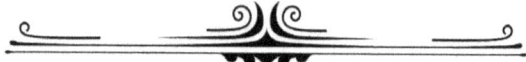

Zen tells us it is important to sit in silence.
Nurses understand they need not always
share their points of view with others.
They know that many times silence is the
best thing they can contribute to a
conversation. Silence shows respect for the
patient who is speaking.

Ethics

Zen's ethics are based on compassion
and wisdom. Zen seeks to lessen
suffering. Nurses ask themselves how
they can best suspend the suffering of
the patients they serve. Sometimes,
assisting the patient to understand
what is going to happen next helps.
Fear is allayed. Other times, teaching a
patient how to compensate for a
weakness alleviates anxiety and worry.

Do No Harm

Zen encourages followers to take only
positive actions. Nurses seek to do no
harm, only good. It is a nurse's nature
to be generous of spirit and disciplined
to do what is honest and right.

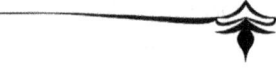

Meditation

Zen uses meditation as a way of clearing the mind to find answers. Nurses require quiet times to focus their thoughts on what needs to happen for the patient. Meditation helps nurses be more aware and rested so they can act in the best interest of a patient.

Thoughts

Zen tells us to look deeply into each
day. Sometimes the future for a patient
looks sad. Out of depths of despair,
nurses are able to create some good
times for patients and their families.
Nurses view each day with a measure
of hope, full of potential, not
necessarily for the future, but simply
for the day at hand.

Seeing the Oneness

Zen is about oneness of the universe.
Zen cares not how many degrees we
have or books we've read. Rather, Zen
cares about the spirit we will be when
we die and all worldly things fall away
from us. Nurses learn patients are
pretty much alike despite the
differences in their education, race,
social status and religion. Where
others see diversity, nurses see
oneness. Because nurses have come to
understand the cohesion of the
universe, they bond with patients.

Impermanence

Zen recognizes the impermanence of
life. Nothing lasts forever. We must be
open to all possibilities. Nurses see
patients change. Some change for the
better and others change for the worse.
Nurses are ready for either situation.

Every Day is a Good Day

Zen teaches each day can be good. We must strive to make it so. Nurses create an atmosphere where much can be enjoyed. Sometimes a little good is good enough. We can be satisfied with a little progress and walk away with satisfaction, knowing we gave the day our best.

Strength from Nature

Zen says we should be one with and draw our strength from nature. There are days nurses feel they will crumble under the pressure of their job duties. Knowing this, nurses may take short breaks away from patient units to places where they can meditate. There is no better place than one with a view of trees. Trees are among nature's strongest and most agile creations with great ability to sway and stay despite winds and bad weather. Nurses can tap into the power of trees to renew themselves. Then, nurses can let patients lean on them for strength.

Courage

Zen tells us courage helps us walk
through whatever we fear. Nurses help
patients make their way through many
trials up to and through death. A nurse's
calmness born of knowledge, experience,
and wisdom helps a patient meet the
unfamiliar without fear.

Always Thinking

Zen is a thinking person's philosophy.
Nurses cluster cues from what the patient
says and what the patient does. Nurses
determine the patient's areas of weakness
and finds ways to resolve them.

Weaknesses

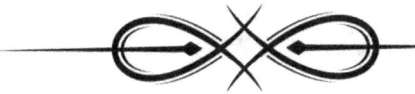

A Zen koan is a puzzling question
without a specific answer. One Zen
koan asks why mankind is weak.
Nurses realize there is value in
understanding our individual
weaknesses. Nurses' insights into their
own weaknesses allow them to
understand patients' vulnerabilities
and thereby, be less judgmental and
more accepting of patient frailties.

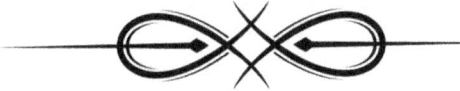

Called by Name

It is written we shall all be called by name. When patients feel lost and alone in the impersonal stream of events in our healthcare system, nurses surprise them by smiling and calling them by name. Nurses want patients to know their uniqueness matters. Nurses recognize that calling patients by name makes patients feel respected and more comfortable.

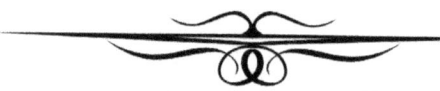

Touch

Zen says to be aware of each other's needs.
Often in quiet stillness, a nurse reaches
out to touch a patient. Nurses know touch
can channel energy from themselves to
patients. A nurse's touch can pull a listless
patient suddenly into a healing encounter.
A smile can make someone's heart feel
better and their body repair.

Persistence

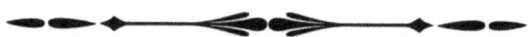

Zen is persistent. Likewise, nurses do
not give up on anyone. Over and over
nurses provide treatment, hoping a
patient may feel better and be made
more comfortable.

Language

Zen might ask what language God speaks. Nurses answer that God's voice is heard in the everyday actions of people caring for one another. Nurses follow the universal tenet of all religions: Do good. Do no harm.

The Growing Edge

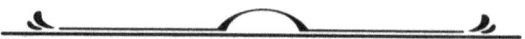

Zen teaches us that we continue to grow on life's journey to the end. Nurses find they learn more and better ways to provide care by going through experiences with patients. Each encounter may teach the nurse another way of practice that can be used to help future patients. That is the nature of the growing edge. The skills of nurses keep growing during their lifelong journeys.

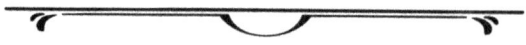

Reflection

Zen says reflection cultivates knowledge. Reflection is an important facet of learning. Patients tell nurses their feelings when they go through medical procedures. By reflecting on patients' experiences, nurses capture the knowledge to better prepare other patients who will undergo similar procedures. Research has shown that better prepared patients have improved recovery rates.

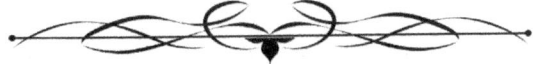

Listening

Zen teaches us to be fully present for each other. Nurses understand listening to another requires turning off all the busyness going on in their own minds if they are to fully hear what is on a patient's mind. Many times nurses stop attending to all the IV lines and other high-tech equipment and intentionally position themselves where patients can see and hear that the nurses are there for them. Good nursing care may just be this listening presence.

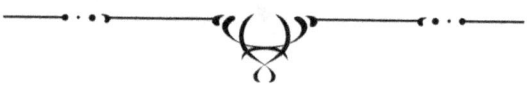

Dialogue

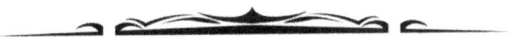

Zen tells us life is meant to be a two-way street paved between one person and another. There should be no domination of one person over the other. Some medical people preach. Nurses' dialogue. Nurses have a habit of listening to patients' wishes and involving patients in their own healthcare decisions. The nurse's role is to support whatever choices a patient makes about their life and death.

Humility

Zen teaches there is much to gain when
a person forgets about him or herself.
Nurses find that if they put their own
thinking aside and take into account
the broader views of other healthcare
workers caring for the same patients, a
better plan for how to get patients
more comfortable often results.
Because nurses can be humble and let
ideas other than their own come into
play, care plans become more broadly
suited for patients and bring about
better outcomes.

Saying Nothing

Zen recognizes silence may be the best contribution a person can make to a conversation. Nurses can sense when patients think best without more discussion. Nurses may sit for long periods with patients and not say a word. Such silence speaks volumes.

Understanding Where Others Are

Zen seeks to understand where others are in their journeys. Nurses who are wise realize they do not have total control over situations. When bad things happen, like a patient falling and getting hurt or a patient crying out in pain, a wise nurse does not lay blame. Instead, the nurse seeks to understand what has happened so similar unfortunate situations may be prevented from occurring. Nurses are committed to assessing people and circumstances.

Sanctity of Daily Life

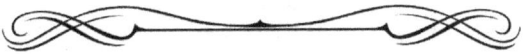

Zen reminds us that everyday life is sacred. Nurses understand their daily care of patients is spiritually driven. They know life is about doing that which, if we were in the patient's condition, we would want done for us.

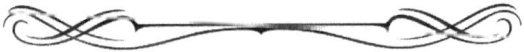

Connectedness

Zen does not require great works. It asks for connectedness. Nurses connect wherever, whenever and with whomever they are assigned. They learn what they can and will do for patients. These experiences in connectedness help nurses know themselves better.

Zen: A Living Philosophy

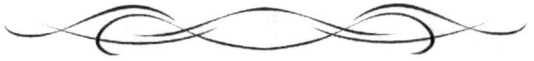

Zen is not an end unto itself. It is a pathway that nurses naturally follow to guide their professional attitudes and nursing practices. Nurses know that every act they perform and every conversation they have should be representative of the person they have chosen to be.

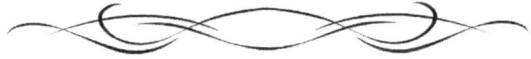

Miracles

Zen may ask why miracles happen.
Nurses would answer, "Because the
universe calls for such miracles." Some
miracles are dependent on nursing
care. Nurses are miracle workers.

Meaningful Work

Zen says work should not be a series of meaningless tasks but rather the process of creating something anew. Nurses work hard each day to create enthusiasm and new strengths in the patients for whom they care. Nurses work in meaningful ways on many levels to help patients, families and communities, and also to advance nursing knowledge and practice.

Following Life's Paths

Those who follow the Zen philosophy
believe it is important to pursue
pathways that present to them. Often
nurses are in just the right place at just
the right time to be able to help patients
understand what is happening to them
in changing healthcare systems.

Giving and Receiving Love

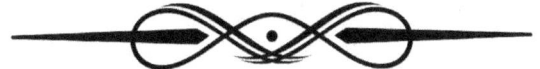

Zen would say to love oneself
unconditionally and also to love one
another: this is the highest of gifts. Nurses
help patients achieve this self-actualization.

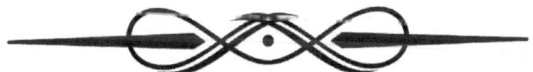

Paying Attention to the Needs of Others

Ordinary life is the heart of Zen. Nurses understand this and pay attention to the commonplace needs of patients. Caring for others is "living Zen."

Everything in Its Time

In Zen, there is an understanding that everything comes along as it does for reasons unknown to us. Nurses come along at just the right time for many patients. Patients frequently remark their lives would have been impossible to live without nurses.

Lightening the Burden of Anger

Zen reminds us that anger corrodes the vessel in which it resides rather than the person for whom the anger is intended. Nurses listen when patients vent their frustrations. Without judging, nurses support patients when they unleash their anger. In this way, patients' burdens are lightened and more of patients' energies may be directed toward healing.

Then and Now

Zen urges us to focus on what is now,
not always be wishing for something
more. Nurses find their working
conditions are not always just as they
would like. But nurses transcend their
often spartan surroundings and
perform extraordinary acts of
professionalism.

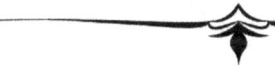

Unsettled Matters

Zen is comfortable with unsettled matters, realizing life is like leaves scattered this way and that...beautiful, with many variations. Nurses are faced with many varied tasks at the start of each shift. They identify and act first on that which is most important.

Inside Out

Zen takes our accomplishments lightly.
Our endeavors are fleeting. Zen knows
what really counts is not who we are on
the outside, but who we are inside.
Who we become, lasts. Nurses become
doers of good.

Forgiveness

Zen says forgiveness is a virtue. Nurses understand we can forgive each other when we can face our own weaknesses and forgive ourselves. Nurses help patients accept themselves and their illnesses.

Thankfulness

Zen tells us that to be grateful is good. Being thankful is a virtue. Nurses walk the halls with extra "thank-yous" in their pockets. Nurses know the "thank-yous" will make patients feel respected.

Relationships

Zen tells us that if we want to feel truly
human, we must reach out to others.
Nurses understand that our human
relationships define us. Nurses are
always reaching out to patients and
drawing family members and friends
into the healing circle.

Now

In Zen, there is no past or future, only now. The past is gone. The future can only be imagined. Nurses know that at each moment they can make a difference now in the life of a patient.

Art of Professionalism

Zen urges us to focus on the present. Nurses face conditions each day that could be better...better staffing, more supplies, etc. Rather than make such concerns the center of their attention, nurses transcend what is, and fill each ordinary day with extraordinary professionalism and kindness.

Memory

Zen reminds us we are all part memory.
Tucked inside each of us, there is a
record of people and places we've met
along our lifetimes. Nurses understand
that patients' memories sometimes are
sorrowful. Nurses can attend to patients'
sadness by listening to stories of their
lives. Many times, a nurse allowing
opportunities for sadness to come out
relieves the pressure of the patient
keeping it inside.

Explanations

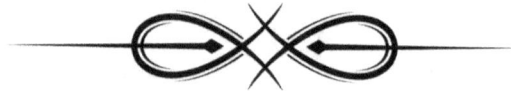

Zen understands that the unknown often
scares us. Nurses make a habit of talking
to patients about their conditions, tests
and treatments. In this way, nurses give
patients maps--concrete ways--in which to
focus their days instead of intangible
fears of the unknown.

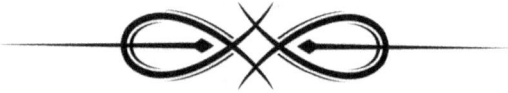

Trust

Zen asks us to trust the universe.
Patients trust nurses. This unspoken
arrangement with patients allows
nurses to reach into the guarded places
where patients keep their innermost
thoughts. Nurses hold patients'
thoughts in a sacred space and do not
reveal secrets.

Passageways

Zen reminds us that birth and death are just passages. Nothing really comes or goes. Rather, all things are transformed. Nurses are present to help patients pass through birth and death.

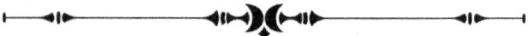

Making Room for Love

Zen knows the angry heart has no
room for love. Nurses encourage
patients to talk about what is annoying
them. After talking with nurses about
their anger, patients often realize that
being angry has prevented love from
reaching them.

How We Listen

Zen reminds us to examine how we listen. A nurse pays attention to a patient's conversation, knowing full well he or she may be hearing a person's last cherished words.

Expectation

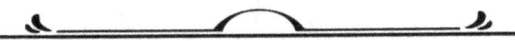

Zen cautions us to not expect life will
give us everything we want. Rather,
life expects something from us. Nurses
work very hard, knowing that society
looks to them to care for others.

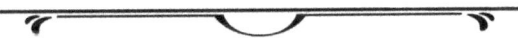

Planes of Existence

Zen tells us a single moment of existence is
not owned by anyone. Each moment resides
in various levels of awareness and in the
thoughts of many people. Nurses seek to
meet patients at the place in each moment
where they dwell.

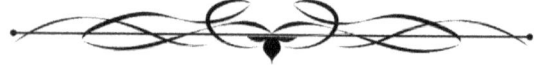

Beneficence

Zen realizes a person may create a good for others. Patients recall nurses who have been great blessings just by the quality of their presence.

Mental Energy

Zen tells us that thoughts are
energy...mental energy. Nurses can
change thoughts into action when they
plan care that helps patients feel better.

Examining Our Lives

Zen tells us that to guide someone else we each must have examined our own life. Nurses know they must take time to contemplate their own place in the world before helping patients examine theirs.

Intention

Zen leads us to know that the very
presence of a person can bring healing.
A nurse's motive is to heal, and this
intention makes healing possible.

Spiritual Guidance

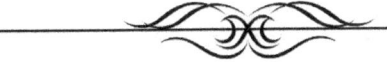

Zen recognizes there are spiritual
guides who divinely inspire people.
Nurses teach patients ways to live
healthier lives.

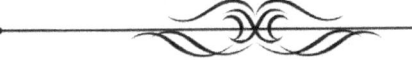

Love & Grace

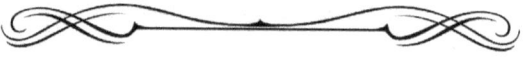

Zen knows love is not what we deserve
but what comes to us from grace.
Nurses help patients know they are
loved and respected. Patients often say
that a nurse has been an unexpected
blessing in their life.

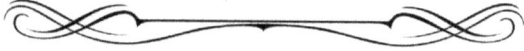

Empathy

Zen says we need to empathize with each other. A nurse says, "I feel for you. I am here to help you."

But for Grace

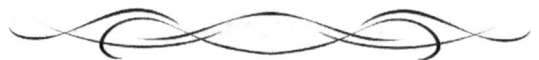

Zen encourages us not to judge by appearances. Nurses do not judge people. Nurses perceive patients as much like themselves. They show understanding and compassion. They realize, "There, but for grace, go I."

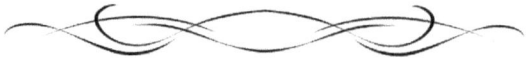

Blame

Zen is not interested in laying blame.
Nurses do not focus on behaviors that led
to an illness. They center their energies
on helping a patient becoming better.

Connectedness

Zen tells us the meaning and purpose
of life is to put our own ego aside and
come to know our connectedness to
everyone and everything in the world.
The nurse puts ego aside, forgetting
about his or her own issues to focus on
what is important to the patient.

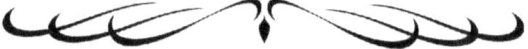

Validating Each Other

Zen says we validate each other
through our interactions. A nurse
confirms a patient's thinking and
perceptions so the patient feels
recognized and whole.

Doing Good

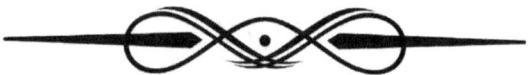

Zen says that doing good is love. The nurse's mode of being in the world is to do good. This love for others' welfare comforts and heals.

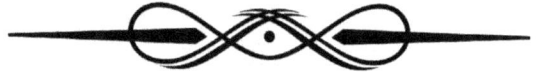

Receptivity

Zen harkens us to be receptive at all times.
Nurses are attentive moment-to-moment.
Because of this watchfulness, nurses pick
up on the feelings of their patients.

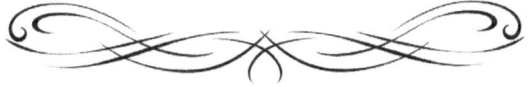

Helping One Another

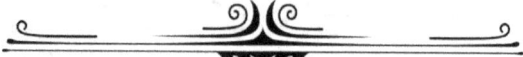

Zen expects us to be open to and to help
one another. Nurses understand they can
help only the patients who let them.

Divine Good

Zen says divine love reveals itself
through the actions of everyday people.
Nurses' actions are the manifestations
of divine good in the world.

Transcending
Everyday Life

Zen tells us to turn our attention away
from everyday life to discover what
truly matters. If we pause and reflect,
we will come to better understand
what is important. Nurses give
patients space and encouragement to
think about their situations in relation
to the meaning of life.

The Enlightened Mind

Zen says a poison arrow cannot lodge itself in an enlightened person. Nurses help patients understand there is more to life than their illness. Believing this, patients find the strength to go forward.

Examining Our Lives

Zen advises us to constantly re-think
the way we do things. Nurses support
patients in their attempts to put aside
unhealthy ways so they can recover.

Learning Life's Lessons

Zen views this life as a place in which a
person learns valuable lessons. Nurses
understand that problems patients face
may turn into opportunities to learn
more about themselves and their
reason for living.

Enjoying Each Moment

Zen says the enlightened person eats when he is hungry and sleeps when he is tired. But unenlightened people think of ten thousand things when they eat and dream of ten thousand things while they sleep. Nurses encourage patients to focus their thoughts on each moment...the pleasure of an enjoyable meal, a lively conversation, a walk outside or a smile sent from someone across the room.

Goodness and Nursing

Zen teaches us we choose what we want to be in this world. Nurses choose nursing because it is intellect, kindness and love strung together in practice.

Temporary Setbacks

Zen tells us things that are seen are temporal and things that are unseen are eternal. Nurses know that patients experience temporary setbacks on the way to becoming who they want to be forever.

We are More Than a Body

Zen believes that when people die their physical bodies disappear from earth. Nurses know that patients are more than bodies. Nurses treat the whole person...body, mind and spirit.

Relaxation, Reflection & Recovery

The art of Zen lies in relaxation, reflection and recovery of strength. Nurses place importance on making quiet times where patients can relax and reflect, spending time with their own thoughts. Nurses know that uninterrupted quiet time allows a patient a space to sort through and discard unnecessary worry.

Divined Meetings

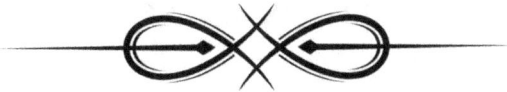

Zen believes there is a reason people meet. Nurses often help patients connect with the healthcare personnel who can best help them with their problems.

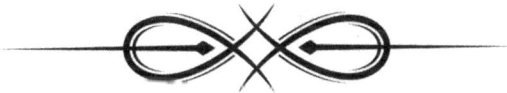

Compassionate Atmosphere

Zen calls on humans to be compassionate.
Healing often manifests itself in the
compassionate, nonjudgmental
atmosphere nurses create.

The Universe of Healing Ways

Zen teaches us we are part of
something greater than ourselves.
Nurses understand they are elements
in the universe of healing ways.

Self-Examination

Zen tells us not to fear when someone
withdraws to examine their life.
Nurses understand that people need
time alone to think and to measure
themselves against the expectations
they have for themselves.

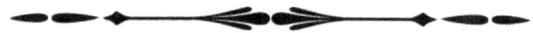

Meditation Time

Zen teaches us that meditation, whether it be for an hour or a day, or 40 days and 40 nights, allows a person to loosen their ties with the earth and turn attention inward to what really counts -- development of their spirit. Nurses respect this process and do not disturb patients as they meditate.

Beyond Our Skin

Zen reminds us that awakening to what is beyond life must occur before we can truly awaken in this life. Nurses already know what many do not: that being of service to others is the most satisfying way to live in this life.

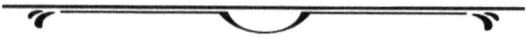

The Starry Sky

Zen cautions us to not be so busy with things of this world that we fail to look up at the stars. Nurses endeavor to place patients where they can commune with and draw strength from nature.

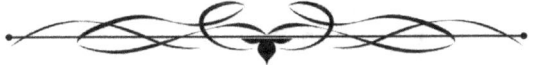

Natural Balance

Zen says do not interfere in the natural balance. Nurses make use of light, fresh air, warmth and music to help patients heal. Florence Nightingale made known these healing ways.

Hopefulness

The Zen mind is one of hopeful
expectancy. Nurses encourage patients to
think positive thoughts and to focus on
the good outcomes for which they hope.

Choosing a Better Future

Zen realizes the future is created by melding what we have learned in the past with our present situation and then looking forward. Nurses discuss with patients what maladies they should leave in their past and what strengths to carry forward. Nurses help patients choose a better future.

Quiet

Zen says the quieter you become, the
more you will hear. It is the pause
between words when Zen is achieved.
The nurse sits down and listens as a
patient unfolds his or her life story.
The nurse serves as a listener. All
patients need someone who will be
quiet and listen to them.

Perception

Zen says perception is everything.
Nurses base their treatments for pain
on what patients say their pain is like.
Nurses trust that the patients'
perceptions are their reality.

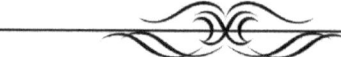

Gentleness

Zen knows that gentleness is better for
the soul than righteousness. A nurse
appreciates that when a patient does
something wrong, gentleness will do
more to heal than reprimand.

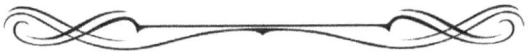

The Truly Evolved Being

Zen knows that enlightened people
display no judgment or bitterness
toward others. Nurses connect without
judging patients. Nurses show no
unpleasantness, even though patients
may show hostility.

Setting Aside Problems

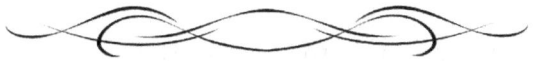

Zen knows that everyday reality is sometimes so harsh that a person has to make a conscious effort to downplay it in order to put together a plan of action. Nurses give patients permission to lay aside their worries about the past so they can gain the strength to go on.

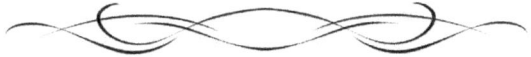

Inner Voices

Zen advises us to shut out the world so
we can hear our own inner voices.
Nurses make conscious efforts to leave
the noise of their job outside a patient's
door to pay attention to the patient's
innermost feelings.

Divine

Zen sees the divine in everyday people. Nurses remind patients they are important to someone and part of the plan of the universe.

Seeing Through Another's Eyes

Zen tells us we cannot be angry with a person when we see things through their eyes. Nurses try to see things from the patient's point of view and then move forward.

Everyday Life

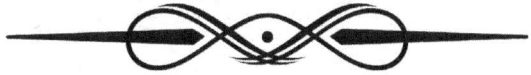

Zen knows that when everyday life is stressful we need to work hard to push troubling circumstances out of our thoughts. A wise nurse is able to set aside ordinary reality and concentrate on what is happening in the patient's world.

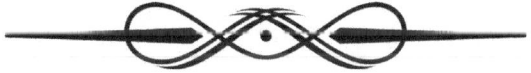

Back and Forth

Zen says we should walk back and forth between our earthly, personal self and our spiritual, divine self. Nurses hold patients' hands as they traverse back and forth.

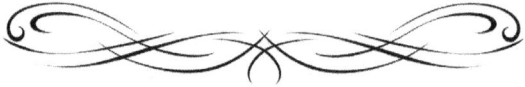

The Quality of Our Journey

Zen reminds us to recognize our life as part of a divinely orchestrated universe. A nurse helps patients know that it is the quality of the journey not the length of the journey that counts.

Time Passing By

Zen operates within two levels of time. One is kronos, the clock time that guides our lives. The other is kairos, which is deeper than just minutes ticking by. Kairos is timeless time -- time that stands still while we get lost deeply engrossed in what we are doing. Nurses encourage patients to get lost in good moments, happy memories and thoughtful, hopeful contemplation. Nurses keep track of kronos, allowing patients to enjoy more moments of kairos.

Doorway to Another World

Zen reveals there is a doorway to another world. Nurses hear patients talking to people who have gone through the portal. Patients say they see and hear people of another world welcoming them to cross over.

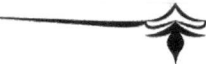

Life & Death

There is a thin veil between life and death. Nurses who care for the dying are holding the hands of people for whom the veil has been lifted. Nurses are privileged to be present at this juncture.

About the Author

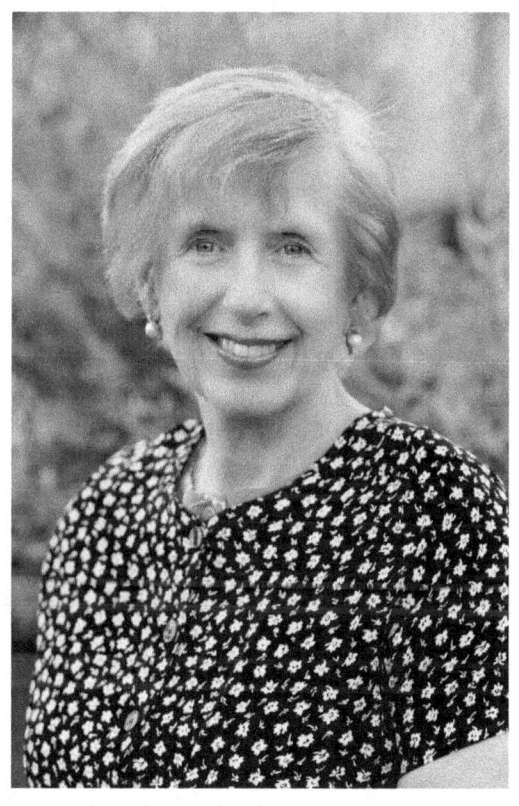

Susan L. Schoenbeck

Susan L. Schoenbeck has been a nurse for more than forty years, working in ICUs, emergency rooms, rehabilitation units, and long-term care administration. She has taught in college nursing programs and has mentored graduate students. Her work has been published in many peer-reviewed journals.

In her books, *Heaven and Angels, The Final Entrance: Journeys Beyond Life* and *Near-Death Experiences: Visits to the Other Side,* Schoenbeck reports experiences of patients who had out-of-body and near-death events. She wrote *Good Grief: Daily Meditations* to meet the bereavement needs of families and friends who lost loved ones.

Schoenbeck lives in Portland, Oregon, where she teaches nursing at Walla Walla University—Portland Campus. She is an oblate of the Holy Wisdom Monastery, which follows the Rule of Benedict.

As an accomplished writer, Schoenbeck has had manuscripts published in journals which attract the attention of physicians and nurses from around the globe. She has also written health care pamphlets directed toward the general public. Schoenbeck served as editor of *Nursing Innovations*, a publication highlighting contemporary accomplishments in nursing.

Schoenbeck is the recipient of many honors including the Universal Voice Award, the Ron Taylor Teaching Excellence Award and state nurse of the year. Schoenbeck is also a recognized speaker and is much in demand for lectures on near-death and deathbed experiences and spiritual care. Her audiences vary, from health-care professionals interested in life's final stages to community groups gathered primarily to hear stories relating to edge-of-death encounters. Her speaking engagements include personal appearances as well as television and audio programs.

In all of her writing and in her speaking engagements, Schoenbeck draws on her many years of clinical nursing, as well as reports from others relating to the edge of death. Her areas of specialty practice are bereavement, counseling the dying and their families, and nursing personnel as they face, in her words, "death as a life event." She is past president of a chapter of Sigma Theta Tau, the International Honorary Society for Nurses. Schoenbeck is a member of the International Association for Near-death Studies. She is currently a board member of the Northwest Association for Death Education and Bereavement Support.

To learn more about Susan Schoenbeck, or where to purchase books, visit: www.susanschoenbeck.com.

www.ingramcontent.com/pod-product-compliance
Lightning Source LLC
Chambersburg PA
CBHW070701290526
45790CB00001B/405